Viroj
Wiwanitkit

Point
of care
testing

iMedPub

Title   ***Point of care testing*** *by Viroj Wiwanitkit*

ISBN-13:   978-1466256958
ISBN-10:   1466256958

Cover design and Layout: Elizabeth Log
                            elizbeth.log@hotmail.com

Publisher   **Internet Medical Publishing**
                info@imedpub.com
                http://imedpub.com/

First edition   **2011**

Viroj
Wiwanitkit

Point of care testing

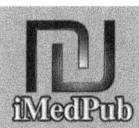

iMedPub

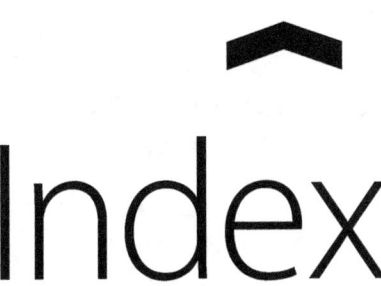

Index

Introduction to point of care **testing**   3

What's the point of care testing?   4

Quality cycle for POCT   5

The factors deteriming the success of POCT system[3]   6

Setting of the new POCT system in a hospital[1]   7

Advantage of the implementation of POCT
system in real clinical practice[1-7]   10

Where can the new POCT system can be
implemented and used?   11

References   13

Basic knowledge on the point of care testing **analyzer** 15

What is the POCT analyzer? 16

Management of the POCT analyzer[1-8] 19

In brief there are many factors to be concerned[1-2] 21

Basic principle of laboratory analysis
by POCT tool[/2] 21

What to be done in case that there is a problem
with the POCT analyzer 23

References 24

Laboratory information management system for point of care **testing** 25

General knowledge on laboratory information
management system[1] 26

Computer laboratory information management
system for point of care testing[2-4] 28

Important software for POCT computer laboratory
information management system [1-5] 29

The implementation of the POCT computer laboratory
information management system 29

Safety of the POCT computer laboratory information
management system 30

References 31

Preanalytical phase for point of care **testing** 33

Introduction to preanalytical phase 34

Request of the laboratory analysis[2-3] 34

Specimen collection[6]   35
Error in preanalytical phase of POCT[2, 9]   36
References   38

Analytical phase for point of care **testing**   39

Introduction to analytical phase[1]   40
Analytical technique[2]   41
Qaulity control for analytical phase for POCT system[1, 3 - 4]   41
Error in analytical phase of POCT[7 - 8]   42
References   43

Postanalytical phase for point of care **testing**   45

Introduction to postanalytical phase   46
Report of laboratory result[1]   46
Interpretation of laboratory result[1]   47
Qaulity control for postanalytical phase
for POCT system[3 - 4]   48
Waste management   48
Error in postanalytical phase of POCT [6 - 7]   48
References   49

Point of care testing for blood glucose **study**   51

Blood glucose[1]   52
Point of care testing for blood glucose study   53

Other point of care testings for diabetic care[1-2]   55
References   56

Point of care testing for lipid **study**   57

Blood lipid[1-2]   58
Point of care testing for lipid study   59
References   61

Point of care testing for coagulation **study**   63

Blood coagulation system   64
Problem on blood coagulation   64
POCT for coagulation study   65
References   67

Blood gas analysis and oint of care **testing**   69l

Introduction to blood gas analysis   70
POCT for arterial blood gas analysis   71
References   73

Point of care testing for thyroid **disease** 75

Introduction to thyroid disease   76
Why the POCT is useful for management
of thyroid disease?   77
POCT tools for thyroid diseases   78
References   79

X

Preface

Point of care testing (POCT) is a new concept in laboratory medicine that is widely used at present. It is the new advent that helps ease medical care in the present day. The knowledge on the POCT medicine is very important and necessary for the general practitioner. In this specific book, the author summarizes, presents and discusses on the concept of POCT, its importance and examples of important POCT tools.

Professor: Viroj Wiwanitkit

March 2011

Introduction to point of care testing

What's the point of care **testing**?

Point of care testing (POCT) is a new concept in laboratory medicine that is widely used at present. Basically, the laboratory investigation is one of the two main tools of the physicians for management of a patient, the laboratory investigation and drug therapy. The aim of the laboratory investigation is to diagnosing of the abnormality of the patient. The investigation in medicine has a very long history. At first, it was the role of the general physician to perform such test. However, when there are a lot of advent and influx of huge workload to the physician, the role is changed to be taken by the medical scientist or medical technologist.

The setting of the specific medical laboratory in the hospital has been done for centuries. The laboratory takes the responsibility in performing the test according to the medical orders. The specific branch of medicine, clinical pathology is developed at that time.

Focusing on the present laboratory investigations, there are two main forms as the followings

1. Investigation at the central laboratory

    Investigation at the central laboratory is the investigation that is performed in the central laboratory of the hospital. This is the classical approach. The specimens are collected form the ward or clinic and passed to the central laboratory for laboratory analysis then the results are reported back from the central laboratory.

2. Investigation at bedside

    Investigation at bedside is the usage of simple laboratory investigation at the bedside. The physicians or in-charge nurses perform some simple tests for rapid assessment of the patients' status. The examples of those tests are hematocrit, urinalysis, etc. This helps fasten the laboratory analysis process.

Table 1. Comparison between investigation at the central laboratory and investigation at bedside[1].

Aspects	bedside	Central laboratory
Speciemen collection	By attending physician or in - charge nurse	By medical technologist
Specimen transportation	This step is skipped, fasten the overall process	Require
Laboratory analysis	By physician in charge, might lack for good quality control process	Has to follow the laboratory guidelinea and standards
Result reporting	No need for specific system since the result is at site	Require

The newest concept, Point of care testing (POCT), is the concept that has just been introduced for a few years. POCT concept is based on both described concepts and this hybrid seems to be a really useful technology in laboratory investigation at present. The POCT concept used these followings

1. Use of an-easy to use analytical tool at the bedsite

2. Canbe simply performed at bedside by physician and in-charge nurse

3. The newest concept is the most convenience technique that can be use by the patient ownself. The good example is the self blood glucose monitoring.

4. There is a guideline and standard for quality management of the labotatory analysis. This is usually by help of the central laboratory in the hospital.[2]

   • In summary the POCT means

   • The newest laboratory investigation system

   • The use of new advanced analyzer tool to serve the analysis at bedsite or site of care of the patient

   • The system that can be flexible for usage at anywhere

   • However, the most direct definition can be "THE SYSTEM OF LABORATORY INVESTIGATION THAT IS PERFORMED AT THE SITE OF MEDICAL CARE"

Quality cycle for **POCT**

Basically, there is a concept namely laboraoty cycle in clinical pathology. This concept describes for the phase of laboratory investigation. Three main phases, pre-analytical phase, analytical phase and post-analytical phase are mentioned. This is the very basic rule that everyone who works in the medical laboratory has to recognize.

Focusing on the new POCT concept, the quality cycle can also be applied.

1. Pre-analytical phase

   This means the phase from specimen collection to the analysis. The sample transportation and preparation are also included into this phase. However, for the POCT technology, the transportation and preparation of specimen are usually skipped.

2. Analytical phase

   This is the actual analytical process. For POCT, this is done at site. The problem of quality control can be corrected if there is the complete usage of POCT quality management system that requires the quality control by the central laboratory.

3. Post-analytical phase

   This is the phase after the actual analysis. This includes the validation of the result and the reporting system. For POCT, this phase is very short since the result can be abruptly displayed.

However, there are also some important concerns for the investigation based on the POCT system.

1. Pre-analytical phase

   • Might easily omit the rechecking of the patient identification

   • Usually lack for the control of the laboratory request form

2. Analytical phase

   • Quality control can be missed if the practitioner overlook it

   • Post-analytical phase

3. Validation of the result can be easily missed

   • Might lack the complete result data record

   • Might pose the problem for charging of the laboratory cost

The factors deteriming the success of POCT system[3]

There are many factors determining the success of POCT system. Briefly, it can be demonstrated as the followings.

1. The medical personnel at ward have to have good knowledge and attitude to the system since they are the main users.

2. The laboratory personnel have also to have good knowledge and attitude to the system since they have to support the system especially for the quality management.

3. The hospital administrator has to set the specific fund for the system

4. The new POCT tools have to be available.

5. It will be better if there is a specific laboratory information management system for supporting on the POCT system within the hospital.

It should be noted that all factors are required. Lack for only one factor can result in the incompleteness of the system and this mean the unsuccess.

In addition, there are more concerns to be addressed as the followings.

1. The system has to be ongoing. It is easily said that "the show must go on". When the system is implemented, there should be a system to support and maintain its function. Implementation is important but the maintenance is more important.

2. Tool is tool. The important factor is the human factor. Since medical personel is the actual user, there has to be a good preparation for all users in the system. The quality system can be used but it will be useless if the practitioner do not recognize and follow it.

3. There must be the maintenance cost. The hospital administrator has to think this before implementation. No maintenance means high risk for error and the downgrading of the system.

4. The hospital administrator has to have a good knowledge and attitude to the system because he/she has to be the director of the implement system.

5. As noted, the computational information management system is very important. It might be expensive but it seems to be a cost-effective apparatus to help reach the success of the system. Considering the cost-utility, the using of the computational information management system seems to be appropriate.

6. When the system is implemented, it has to be actuall used. The strict practice according the guideline and rule is required.

Setting of the new POCT system in a **hospital**[1]

As already noted, it has to be carefully considered before setting of a new POCT system in the hospital. There are many reasons.

- The system is expensive.

- The system has to be long run.

- The system needs the attention by the practitioner.

- The system requires cost.

However, to reach on the best service, it is no doubt that we should turn to the implementation and usage of the new POCT system. The reasons include:

- Fast service means good service

- Reduction of the turnaround also means increase the satisfaction of the patient

- Reduction of step means decrease error in overall process

- Collaboration between medical personnel means good collaboration within the hospital.

Hence, it is no doubt to set the POCT system in the hospital. However, the present question can be "How can I set such system?" This can be easily answered. Please follow these instructions.

To set a new POCT system in a hospital, there has to be a good preparation. Indeed, to do anything, the preparation is required. Good preparation means success. Basically, to set a new POCT system in a hospital, the concept of setting of the central laboratory within the hospital can be followed. The details are hereby shown.

1. The first step is the situation analysis. This means you have to know your own current status before further performing anything. This means you have to get all data on all aspects of your laboratory. Workplace and workflow analysis have to be done. The necessary things to be known include

   - Present workflow chart

   - This is very important since this means the actual thing that actually existed. This helps plan set the proper and most fit system.

   - Present workload

   - This is very important since we have to provide the system that can serve the present workload and must also serve the future situation.

   - Labor

     This means know the actual number of the personnel involving and working on the newly implemented system.

   - Apparatus and tolls

     Survey on the present apparatus and tools is needed. This helps us see the picture and need for new POCT tool. This also plan allocating the new POCT tool to the correct place.

   - Place dimension

     This is helpful to set the allocation plan of the newly implemented POCT system.

   - Commnunication

     This is helpful to determine the need of implement of new communication, information technology, for supporting the newly implemented POCT system.

   - Connection

     This means the support and collaboration with outside panels. This can be helpful data for future expansion of the system to extrahospital network.

- Fund and cost

  This is really important thing to know. This helps make decision on what to pay first and what to implement first.

2. When the first step, the situation analysis, is ready. All gathering data has to be used. The discussion among the group of hospital admintration board is requied. This means the step to make decision on implementation. Also, if the decision is made, it has to be already have a plan to select the most appropriate system. This is really the policies making step.

3. When the hospital administration board has a clead decision to set and implement the new POCT system, the next step is to prepare for the setting. This means the preparation for completeness of all things to hold the newly implemented POCT syste. The things to be done include:

   - Declaration on the policy

   - Broadcasting of the vision and mission

   - Set the timeframe and corresponding working group

   - Knowledge settlement to all units within the hospital

   - Traning session for all medical personnel

   - Making agreement between units within the hospitals

   - Clarifying the role of the ward and laboratory unit

   - It should be noted that this step is the heart of the success of the implementation. The hospital administrator has to work hard and has to have a good leadership.

4. Then, it is the time to set and implemented the system. The firt trial has to be done. This means the period to see the error and problem. Correction of idenfied errors and problems has to be done. Readjustment of the system is needed.

5. Finally, it is the step of actual using! We have to use and maintain it. The good concept for maintenance is pan-do-check-ack.

   - Plan

     There has to be good plan for management of the implemented POCT system.

   - Do

     "Do" means actual running and working based on the already set plan.

   - Check

     Checking or monitoring of the situation during running the plan has to be done. This means continuous quality improvement too.

   - Act

     If any errors or problems occur, action is required. Although there is no problem, we should have to find the new chance to further improve or develop the system to the better status. It should be noted that the technology never stops hence we have to continuously update.

Advantage of the implementation of POCT system in real clinical **practice**[1-7]

It is no doubt that the POCT concept is the new useful concept in laboratory medicine. As already discussed, it is the hybrid that takes the advantages from laboratory analysis at central laboratory and laboratory analysis at bedside.

If there is a question whether the actual advantage of the POCT system is, the easy answers can be as the followings.

1. Help shorten the laboratory process

    It is accepted that the clascial laboratory process takes a long time. This means the patients have to wait and the physicians also have to wait. What is the problem of waiting? There are many answeres:

    *   Lost of labor cost

    *   Lack for chance to do other things

    *   Some illness will continuously downhill during waiting time

    *   Long waiting time means increase chance or error

    *   Long waiting time means decrease patient satisfactory and this also the basic thing leads to the complaint and sue.

2. Increase the quality of classical investigation at bedsite

    The implementation of the POCT system helps correct the basic problems of classical investigation at bedside. In an easy word, it helps correct the problem of "quality". To help the reader imagine, the descriptions are

    *   Decrease the error due to poor analytical tool (no standard, under standard)

    *   Decrease the error due to lack of quality control

    *   Decrease the error due to untrained practitioner

        The good example is the increase the quality in using of simple analytical tool, arterial blood gas analyzer. In the past time, the error in using this analyzer at bedside is common and the main reason is the lack for the good quality management problem. Since the result from arterial blood gas analysis is an actual critical parameter, hence, it can seriously affect the patient if the result in not correct.

3. Leads cost effectiveness in using laboratory tool[8]

    The implementation of the new POCT system help reach cost effectiveness in using laboratory tool. Some readers might not understand how cost effectiveness can be received because of the picture of high cost of the system. The answers include.

    *   Reduction in error means reduction of cost for repeated analysis

    *   Reduction in error means reduction of cost that might occur if there is a medical sue problem

- Reduction in error means increase satisfaction and reuse of the service in the future time from the patient

- Reduction in overall turnaround time means increase time to do other things and get new productivity

- Clarification of the exact volume by good recording system help manage the charge and payment in bedsite laboratory analysis

---

Where can the new POCT system can be implemented and **used**?

The POCT system is basically designed to be feasible and flexible. This means the POCT system can be implemented and used in several places. By its names, it is used at point of care or where the patient is.

So it can be applied for these places

- Hospital
  - Out patient clinic (OPD)
  - In patient clinic (IPD)
  - Emergency room (ER)
  - Operation room (OR)
  - Labor room (LR)
  - Intensive care unit (ICU)
  - Cardiac care unit (CCU)
  - Immediate cardiac care unit (ICCU)
- Clinic
- At patient home (self monitoring)
- At emergency car of the hospital
- At community (with health team)
- Anywhere (most ideal)
  - Hence, it can be said that the POCT tool can be applied in all levels of medical service
  - Primary care
  - Secondary care
  - Tertiary care

In additional to the question "Where can the new POCT system can be implemented and used?", another interesting question is "Who can use the new POCT system?"

This question is already partially discussed. The answers can be

- Patient

- This is the most ideal used. Indeed, the concept of present medicine is promoting of the patient to take care his/herself. The implementation of the POCT tool can be an answer. There are many available POCT analyzers that can be used for self-monitoring. The most famous analyzer is the self-moniotring glucometer. This is the basic thing that is recommended for all diabetic patients.

- Medical personnel

  This is the usage in the first development of the POCT tool. Firstly, the laboraoty technician has to well understand the principle of the POCT analyzer. Sometimes, big POCT analyzers are very similar to dry chemistry analyzer and can be adopted for usage in the central laboratory of the hospital. However, the main important group of users is the medical personnel in the ward, physicians and nurses. These medical personnel have to be well trained and effectively use those POCT tools

- Public health personnel

  It is accepted that an important group of people that plays important role in health system is the public health personnel. These workers play important role in primary care unit and rural field work. Also, these workers take important role in pre-hospital care as the rescue team in emergency car.

References

1. Wiwanitkit V. Management of quality in medical laboratory. Bangkok: Chulalongkorn University Press, 2005.

2. Misiano DR, Meyerhoff ME, Collison ME. Current and future directions in the technology relating to bedside testing of critically ill patients. Chest. 1990;97(5 Suppl):204S-214S

3. Schallom L. Point of care testing in critical care. Crit Care Nurs Clin North Am. 1999; 11:99-106.

4. Muller MM, Hackl W, Griesmacher A. Point-of-care-testing--the intensive care laboratory. Anaesthesist. 1999;48:3-8.

5. Kost KJ. Guidelines for point-of-care testing. Improving patient outcomes. Am J Clin Pathol. 1995;104(4 Suppl 1):S111-27.

6. Prince CP. Point-of-care testing. Impact on medical outcomes. Clin Lab Med. 2001;21:285-303.

7. Prince CP. Point of care testing. BMJ. 2001;322:1285-8.

8. Prince CP. Medical and economic outcomes of point-of-care testing. Clin Chem Lab Med. 2002;40:246-51.

Basic knowledge on the point of care testing analyzer

What is the POCT **analyzer**?

This is a very simple question. If we know the concept of the POCT, we can easily tell what the POCT analyzer is.

The POCT analyzer means the tool that

- Is used for POCT work

- Is the generation of analyzer in laboratory investigation system

- Is usually small

- Is designed to serve the analysis at bedsite or site of care of the patient

- Is flexible for usage at anywhere

- However, these properties are in general. Some analyzers might be different. If we try to classify the present existed POCT analyzers in group, we might classify into two main groups. The first group is the tool that is limited for usage by medical or public health personnel. These POCT analyzers are usually complicated, large and hard-to-use. Also, it requires standard quality control process and the referencing of the result is important. The second group is the tool that can be used by anyone. The specific ter, CLEAWAVE, is used for identifying these analyzers. These POCT analyzers are designed for the use at everywhere. It can be used as self-monitoring tool. It can be used in the rural field work. The concept is the serve the need of rapid diagnosis in the limited setting. However, the result from these tools is usually preliminary. It is usually used as a roung tool for screening and following up.

These are the examples of common POCT analyzer at present.

1. Based on the aim of usage

    - For critical care

        - Blood gas analyzer

- For routine care
  - Glucometer
  - Cardiac marker analyzer
  - Blood chemistry analyzer
  - Urinalysis analyzer
  - Hematology analyzer
  - Coagulation profile analyzer
  - Hormone analyzer
- For self-monitoring care
  - Self-monitoring glucometer

2. Based on the place of usage
   - At patient home
     - Self-monitoring glucometer
   - At private clinic
     - Glucometer
     - Cardiac marker analyzer
     - Blood chemistry analyzer
     - Urinalysis analyzer
   - At OPD
     - Glucometer
     - Blood chemistry analyzer
     - Hematology analyzer
     - Coagulation profile analyzer
   - At IPD
     - Glucometer
     - Cardiac marker analyzer
     - Blood chemistry analyzer
     - Urinalysis analyzer
     - Hormone analyzer
     - Hematology analyzer
     - Coagulation profile analyzer

- At ICU
  - Glucometer
  - Blood gas analyzer
  - Cardiac marker analyzer
  - Blood chemistry analyzer
  - Urinalysis analyzer
  - Hematology analyzer
  - Coagulation profile analyzer
- At CCU
  - Glucometer
  - Blood gas analyzer
  - Cardiac marker analyzer
  - Blood chemistry analyzer
  - Urinalysis analyzer
  - Hematology analyzer
  - Coagulation profile analyzer
- At ER
  - Glucometer
  - Blood gas analyzer
  - Cardiac marker analyzer
  - Blood chemistry analyzer
  - Urinalysis analyzer
  - Hematology analyzer
  - Coagulation profile analyzer
- At emergency car
  - Glucometer
  - Cardiac marker analyzer
  - Coagulation profile analyzer
- At rural field work
  - Glucometer
  - Blood chemistry analyzer
  - Urinalysis analyzer

3. Based on the kind of analyzer

- Hematology
  - Cardiac marker analyzer
- Coagulation profile analyzer
  - Clinical chemistry
  - Glucometer
  - Blood gas analyzer
  - Cardiac marker analyzer
  - Blood chemistry analyzer
  - Urinalysis analyzer
- Molecular biology
  - Gene chip
  - PCR-based POCT tool

4. Based on the size of usage

- Pocket size
  - Glucometer
  - Specific POCT meter for monitoring lipid profile
  - Coagulation profile analyzer
- Labtop size
  - Blood gas analyzer
  - Cardia c marker analyzer
  - Blood chemistry analyzer
  - Urinalysis analyzer

Management of the POCT **analyzer**[1-8]

A simple requirement in laboratory medicine is the good management of all laboratory analyzers. Focusing on POCT analyzer, good management is also needed. The process must start at the selection until the maintenance.

1. Selection of the POCT tool

   The first step is the situation analysis as already discussed in the previous chapter. This is required since you have to know your own current status before further performing anything. Complete information on these things are required.

- workflow

- workload

- place

- fund

When we get all information, all gathering data has to be used for decision analysis. These tools should be selected first

- answet the present workload

- fit to the place

- affordable

The further consideration is on the efficacy of the POCT. The concern is based on the basic laboratory medicine principle. These efficacy of every POCT has to be considered and satistifed before final selection

- sensitivity

- specificity

- accuracy

- repeatability

- reproducibility

2. Allocation of the POCT tool

   After we can select the proper POCT tool for user, we have to allocate or distribute it for actual user. The easy principles include

   - Allocate to where it is really needed.

   - Allocate to where it is not available

   - Allocate to where it has high workload

     If we use these principles, we can successfully reach the most effective way of usage of POCT analyzers within the hospital

3. Maintenance of the POCT tool

   Every tool has to be maintained. When we use care, we have to maintain it. Hence, it is no doubt that the use of POCT analyzer needs regular maintenance. The maintenance is required because

   - Every tool can has defective when it is prolonged used

   - Every tool can has bias and error when it is prolonged used

However, these are general basic concern. In real usage, there are many factors that determine the success of mamagement of POCT analyzer. It should be noted that the first POCT analyzer of the world is the glucometer. This kind of analyzer has been used for years. Howefer, at the first phase, it lacked for systematic control. No quality assurance was set.

In brief there are many factors to be **concerned**[1-2]

1. The quality of specimen

   Despite the general routine practice of the medical personnel in their daily work, the error in specimen collection can still be detectable (at a high rate). Hence, it is no doubt that if we allow the patient to perform self-monitoring, more problem on the specimen collection can be expected. Hence, the solution is the designing of the most convenient POCT tool to serve the self-monitoring usage purpose. This is the reason for developing of the CLEAWAVE tool that is easy-to-use and practical for the layperson.

2. The quality control of the system is needed. If this step is neglected, the problem can be imagined. Generally, the central laboratory has to take role in quality control of all POCT tool in the hospital. If there is no quality control system and the physician directly use not non standard laboratory result for caring of the patient, the problem in patient care can be seen. For sure, the result from the self-monitoring tool that lack for regular quality control cannot be used as strong clinical evidence for adjustment of the medical treatment regimen.

3. Routinely, the maintenance of the POCT analyzer is needed. This has to be regularly done. However, in some case, the maintenance is not available and this leads to the defect or error of the in use tool. Hence, the regular maintenance program has to be set. The maintenance should be by both central laboratory medical personnel and the specialist from the POCT analyzer company.

4. If the standard POCT information management system is not implemented, the problem of the data collection can be expected. The serious problem on the financial control of the usage of the POCT analyzer has to be kepted in mind since there is no regulatory control system for rechecking. Last but not least, the problem of corruption of the medical personnel on using of the POCT analyzer without the information control is the real story in developing countries.

Basic principle of laboratory analysis by POCT **tool**[/2]

If we talk about the general POCT analyzer, these characteristics can be seen

- Small
- Flexible
- Movable
- Expensive

Everyone who uses the POCT analyzer knows its appearance but only a few users know how it can work.

An interesting characteristic of the POCT analyzer is requirement of very few amount of specimen. Why it requires only a few amount of blood? This is an interesting question to be answered. This is because of the application of the new laboratory technology calling microfluidics.

Briefly, the microfluidics presents these properties

- Based on the principle of biosensor and electronic chip

  Inside the small POCT analyzer that we see, there are many small electronic circuits on electronic frame.

- Based on the flow principle

  The specimen has to be flown. Control of flow director is the basic requirement. The flow has to on the director of the drawn circuit in the electronic frame. We might separate the portion of flow into four parts

  - Plasma separating layer

    Plasma separating layer is the part that is prepared by fiber optic. It is the part that filtrate the blood cell and allow plams for further flow to the plasma reservoir

  - Plasma reservoir

    Plasma reservoir is also the part that is prepared by fiber optic. It is the part that collects the plasma for further reacting with dry reagent.

  - Reagent layer

    Reagent layer is the part containing the dry reagent. This is used for reacting with plasma. Also, at this part, there is the specific indicator for monitoring the reaction.

  - Magnetic tape

    This is the most important part. It is the magnet chip containing the data and command for interpretation and showing of the result on the screen of the POCT analyzer.

- Based on the amplification of signal

  The POCT analyzer uses the amplification of the signal to amplify the detected signal from biosensor unit to result in the laboratory result.

Focusing on step by step on how the POCT analyzer works, it can be briefly explained as the followings:

1. Open of the analyzer. There is usually an open button for electronic opening of overall function of the POCT analyzer.

2. Specimen collection is done. Generally, the specimen is blood. The blood will be sucked at the specimen orifice of the POCT analyzer.

3. The flow system will operate. The forced direct flow as previously explained passing the four important parts occurs.

4. Dry chemistry reaction occurs.

5. Biosensor detects the signal based on the indicator principle.

6. Processing of the data based of amplication of signal by microcomputer.

7. The final result will be displayed on the screen of the POCT analyzer.

8. Some POCT analyzers can print out the result.

9. Overall, the process can be complete within a short turnaround time.

What to be done in case that there is a problem with the POCT **analyzer**

"What to be done in case that there is a problem with the POCT analyzer" is an interesting query. For sure, any laboratory analyzer can have the problem. The corrective action when there is a problem of the POCT analyzer include

- Stop any analysis

- Reanalysis and if the problem still exists, further check

- Check the completeness of the tool. Simply, check for every button and part of analyzer. Whether it is in the correct place is the first thing to check.

- Check for the quality control record

- Check for the maintenance record

- If there is no solution, contact to the medical engineering specialist of the hospital or the POCT company for resolving of the problem

- Don't forget to record any incidence. This is very useful for planning of preventive action and corrective action in the future.

References

1. Wiwanitkit V. Management of quality in medical laboratory. Bangkok: Chulalong-korn University Press, 2005.

2. Wiwanitkit V. Automated clinical chemistry analyzer. Online Video Conferencing, Research Institute of Chemistry. International Center for Chemical Science University of Karachi, Pakistan. 14 February 2007

3. Pugia MJ, Blankenstein G, Peters RP, Profitt JA, Kadel K, Willms T, Sommer R, Kuo HH, Schulman LS. Microfluidic tool box as technology platform for hand-held diagnostics. Clin Chem. 2005;51:1923-32.

4. Srenger V, Stavljenic-Rukavina A, Cvoriscec D, Brkljacic V, Rogic D, Juricic L. Development of laboratory information system--quality standards. Acta Med Croatica. 2005;59:233-9. .

5. Prince CP. Point-of-care testing. Impact on medical outcomes. Clin Lab Med. 2001;21:285-303.

6. Bennett J, Cervantes C, Pacheco S. Point-of-care testing: inspection preparedness. Perfusion. 2000;15:137-42.

7. Carlson DA. Point of care testing: regulation and accreditation. Clin Lab Sci. 1996;9:298-302

8. Jacobs E, Hinson KA, Tolnai J, Simson E. Implementation, management and continuous quality improvement of point-of-care testing in an academic health care setting. Clin Chim Acta. 2001;307:49-59.

Laboratory information management system for point of care testing

General knowledge on laboratory information management **system**[1]

Basically, the laboratory process is a process that has to deal with a lot of information. For clarification, these are the information within the laboratory that needs management

- Patient identification: hospital number, laboratory number

- Cost and price and charge of laboratory investigation

- Quality control data and quality assurance data

- Laboratory result data

Hence, it is no doubt that there are many data to be managed. Previously, the mamangement of laboratory data had to be manually performed. This led to the lost of human resource for managing of the heap of paper works. For sure, there are many problems on manual management on laboraoty data. These are examples of important problems

- Lost of labor

- Lost of time

- Too slow for management

- Easy to have an error

- Hard to have an update information

- Difficult to control the quality of data management

So the question is how to manage such data. The answer can be the simple one that is widely used for management of any large amount of data. The use of computer is the solution that can be applied within medical laboratory.

The usefulness of computer in management of laboratory data include

- Decrease workload to laboratory personnel
- Save time
- Fast
- Reduce error
- Up to date information management
- Easy to control the quality of data management

Hence, it can be seen that the application of computer system is the answer for this story.

The computer system that is specifically used for management of medical laboratory data is called medical laboratory information management system. This system has just been introduced and used in laboratory medicine for about 10 years. After application in clinical pathology, it is widely recognized for its advantage. Indeed, this is an application of computer engineering technology to answer and solve the problem in medicine.

Bascially, the laboraoty information management system has the three main parts.

1. Software

   Software is the computer program for operating, controlling and managing of the laboratory actitives. The focused processed include analytical activity, validation activity, sample tracing activity, sample identifying activity, quality control acitviity, recheck actitivity and data recording activity

2. Hardware

   Hardware is the computer machine for manipulation and processing of data. It has to be run along with the software.

3. Network

   Only software and hardware is not sufficient for management of the laboratory since a) the laboratory is a large unit, b) there are many analyzers, c) the laboratory has to serve the whole hospital hence interface between laboratory unit and other units is required. The soluliton for solving of the communication problem is the use of the network technology.
   Network technology is the use of the computer system for linkage between units. This can be intranet or internet system. Intranet means linkage between internal units while intranet means linkage to external units. Wire or wireless communication can be selected.

The linkage is usually via the computer network operator and there must be the specific connection site called hub for serving as communication gate way. The computer network system is very helpful for the laboratory with high workload and need on the communication management. In conclusion, the advantage of the computer network system includes

- Manage of the communication within laboratory.

- Manage of the communication to the outside units (inside and outside hospital).

- Can be set as backup system for communication data.

- Control of record on communication.

Computer laboratory information management system for point of care testing[2 - 4]

In the previous day, the computational laboratory information management system meant the specific computer system within the laboratory. This means the limitation of its usage. However, the present concept expands the dimension of usage of computer for information management of the laboratory. The present concept makes use for the computer system for both activities within and outside the medical laboratory.

The examples of such activities include:

- Laboratory request at ward

- Laboratory analysis in the medical laboratory

- Laboratory result reporting

- Quality control management

- Quality assurance system

- Remote site laboratory management

- Telemecine application

Hence, it can be said that the computatitonal laboratory management system has a number of applications and usefulness.

Focusing on the use for information management in POCT science, we call the specific system as POCT computer laboratory information management system. Its specific characteristics are described below:

1. Software

   Specific software is needed for POCT system. There are several available softwares at present. The administrator of the laboratory should carefully select the best software for their laboratories.

2. Hardware

   Specific hardware is needed for POCT system. There are several available hardwares at present. The administrator of the laboratory also need for decision makring to have the best software for their laboratories.

3. Network

   Specific network is needed for POCT system. There are several available networks at present. Most are wireless system. The usage of barcode is important for controlling of laboratory requesting, result reporting and quality controlling.

Important software for POCT computer laboratory information management system [1 - 5]

There are many available softwares for POCT computer laboratory information management system. However, those softwares can be categorized as the following categories.

1. Software for quality controlling

   This is the specific software that is designed to serve the quality control service. This is the necessity thing for implementation of the complete laboratory information management system. The nature of the software should be high secure and possible for remote quality controlling.

2. Software for backing up program

   Software is required for backing up program. Since the use of the recording and manipulating of the information and data via computational system, it poses the risk of lost of information in case of abruptly downing of the electricity. The continuous backing up of the information is required as a safety protocols.

3. Software for specimen collection management

   Since the POCT has a short time for specimen collection period, this specific kind of software might not be important.

4. Software for result reporting management

   Since the POCT has a short time for result reporting period, this specific kind of software might not be important.

The implementation of the POCT computer laboratory information management system

As we noted for the importance of the system, it is no doubt that we should implement the POCT computer laboratory information management system if it is affordable. The process is very important. How to implement the computer system is an important query.

This can follow the principle of self examination, situation analysis and decision making as already discussed.

However, there are also some important considerations to be addressed.

- There must be a committee to control the POCT system within the hospital. Within this committee, a subcommittee to control the POCT computer laboratory information management system should also be set.

- Hardware management is needed. There must be an assigned team to maintain and control the hardware. The hardware should be kept in the secure zone within the hospital. It should also be within the medical laboratory.

- Software maintenance is needed. The team to control and update the softwate must also be set.

- The same practice should be used for the network.

- There should be the good maintenance program for the POCT computer laboratory information management system

These are important rules for maintenance:

- A maintenance schedule is required.

- A specific team for maintaining of POCT computer laboratory information management system is required.

- The user has to follow the instruction of the system. The user should not modify or do anything that can destroy or disturb the normal function of POCT computer laboratory information management system.

- The supplier or the company that sell the system must have post-sale service for regular maintenance and upgrading of the POCT computer laboratory information management system.

Safety of the POCT computer laboratory information management **system**

Finally, the safety of the system should be mentioned. As we know, there is no system that has 100 % security. However, we should have preventive and corrective protocols to correspond with any problems.

The possible insecurity include:

- Misuse of the POCT computer laboratory information management system

- Hacking

- Direct destroying of the system such as fire or flood

References

1. Wiwanitkit V. Laboratory information management system. Chula Med J 2000; 44: 61-68

2. Srenger V, Stavljenic-Rukavina A, Cvoriscec D, Brkljacic V, Rogic D, Juricic L. Development of laboratory information system--quality standards. Acta Med Croatica. 2005;59:233-9.

3. Toffaletti J. Wireless POCT data transmission. MLO Med Lab Obs. 2000;32:44-8, 50-1.

4. DuBois JA. Getting to the point: integrating critical care tests in the patient care setting. MLO Med Lab Obs. 2000;32:52-6.

5. Jahn M. Laboratory information systems, Part 2. How well does LIS reach all 4 corners of the lab? MLO Med Lab Obs. 1996;28:53-7.

Preanalytical phase for point of care testing

Introduction to preanalytical **phase**

Preanalytical phase is the first phase within the laboratory cycle. This is a very importhat phase since it is the first step hence any error in this phase can affect the whole process of laboratory analysis.

The concern of preanalytical phase is the basic rule in laboratory medicine. This has to be implemented for the POCT work. Generally, the quality control of the preanalytical phase is required. There are many reports confirming the importance of this phase. Many reports show the high rate of error in this phase. For example, Wiwanitkit studied the situation in an ISO certified laboratory and found that there was a very high rate of errors[1]. This can reflect the need for preanalytical quality control. However, there is no specific report on the preanalytical error in the POCT system. However, it is expected to be lower than normal laboraoty process since there is a significant reduction of preanalytical process in the POCT system.

However, due to the fact that the medical personnel at ward, OPD or remote site are the main personnel who perform the specimen collection in the preanalytical phase, the control of the competency means control of quality. There is a need for collaboration between laboratory personnel and non-laboratory personnel to develop a specific preanalytical quality control program for the implemented POCT system,

Request of the laboratory **analysis**[2 - 3]

Similar to general laboratory investigation, the request of the laboratory is still required for the POCT system. This means that there has to be a control system for requesting. Generally, the one who takes responsibility for laboratory request is the physician. However, for the POCT, some tools with CLEWAVE can be performed by non physicians. Nevertheless, the rule of laboratory request should be followed. The rational laboratory request is required to fulfille the quality assurance of POCT system.

Basicall, the two indications of the general laboratory investigations include

- There is an indication.
- There is no contraindication.
- Based on these principles, the laboratory request for POCT analysis can be effectively done.

These are the good examples.

- For screening purpose
- Use of glucometer for screening of diabetes mellitus
- For diagnostic purpose
- Use of cardiac marker test for diagnosis of acute myocardial infarction
- For following up purpose
- Use of coagulation test for following up of the patient on anticoagulation therapy

However, it should be noted that the use of POCT significantly reduce the time hence there is usually no laboratory request form. This means lack of evidence for rechecking. If there is no good computer laboratory information management system, it is very hard to check for the use of POCT tool. [4-5] This means

- Lack of control of cost and charge
- Lack of control of laboratory record
- Lack of control of medical record
- Lack of control of nurse record

Hence, it should be kept in mind that the user of the POCT analyzer has to make a complete record to be evidence of good practice. In case that there is an implemented POCT computer information management system, the problem can be reduced and rechecking is feasible. However, this system is based on barcode. Hence, there is still a requirement to get good collaboration from the practitioner on using of the barcode.

Specimen **collection**[6]

Specimen collection is the core process in laboratory analysis. Since the laboratory analysis means the process of analysis of collected specimen from human body for further clinical interpretation. If there is no specimen collection, there is no laboraoty analysis.

The first thing to be say is the general principle of laboratory specimen collection. The requirement is the strict practice according to the clinical pathology principle. First, all collections must be based on the general medical ethics principle. The important rule is "First do no harm" and the second rule is the "informed consent"[7]

Both menionted principles have to be strictly followed. This means the legal and correct practice in the procedure.

Focusing on the POCT system, the widely used specimens include blood and urine. For blood specimens, there are two kinds that are widely used.

- Capillary blood sample

  This is a very basic sample for many POCTmeter at present. It is the most widely used blood specimen in the POCT system.

- Arterial blood sample

  This is specifically used for arterial blood gas analysis.

Focusing on the medical procedures for specimen collections, the important procedures are hereby described.

1. Capillary blood sample collection

   The site is usually at the finger tip. It is advised to puncture at the middle or ring finger of the non dominant hand. The cleansing agent is alcohol. The puncture can be performed by blade, lancet or small needle. Also, there is a specific capillary puncture pen at present, however, the cost is high and might not be affordable in resource limited setting.

2. Arterial blood sample collection[8]

   This is the specific specimen collection that has to be performed by the physician. Since this is considered a harmful technique, there is a need to monitor the procedure and post procedure complication. The site for collection of arterial blood smaple is the arterial pulse at the wrist. The Allen's test to checking for collateral circulation has to be performed before actual practice of blood collection. The septic technique, usage of providone iodine as cleansing agent at skin is required. The glass or specific designed plastic syringe can be selected as collection tube.

Error in preanalytical phase of **POCT**[2, 9]

Similar to general laboratory investigation, the error within the preanalytical phase of PCOT system can be expected. The possible errors include:

- Misidentification of the patient

  This is very common and can be expected. Since there is short time for specimen collection and lack for the good rechecking system. Hence, it is advised to gently recheck and reidentify before performing any specimen collection for POCT system.

- Incorrect specimen collection technique

  The incorrect speciemen collection technique might be expected in the practitioners with low experience. The good examples are the squeezing of caplliray blood sample, venous puncture during arterial blood collection, etc.

  It can be seen that the error in this phase is usually random error which is due to human factor.

To reduce the error, a good quality control is needed for preanalytical phase of POCT system. The principle of prenalaytical quality control for POCT system include:[10-11]

- Increased awareness of the practitioner

- Competency testing

- Rechecking rule as a method for patient identification

- Barcode technology

- Good clinical practice

- Good traning for specimen collection procedure

- Preventinve action setting

- Corrective action setting

- Incident reporting

Finally, it should be noted that the careful practice is the heart for quality management in preanalytical quality control in POCT system.

References

1. Wiwanitkit V. Types and frequency of preanalytical mistakes in the first Thai ISO 9002:1994 certified clinical laboratory, a 6 - month monitoring. BMC Clin Pathol. 2001;1:5.

2. Wiwanitkit V. Quality management in medical laboratory process. Bangkok: Chulalongkorn University, 2005

3. Wiwanitkit V. Screening tests in laboratory medicine: interesting tests and rational use. Chula Med J 2001; 45: 1031-1038.

4. Wiwanitkit V. Laboratory information management system. Chula Med J 2000; 44: 61-68

5. Nichols JH, Bartholomew C, Brunton M, Cintron C, Elliott S, McGirr J, Morsi D, Scott S, Seipel J, Sinha D. Reducing medical errors through barcoding at the point of care. Clin Leadersh Manag Rev. 2004;18:328-34.

6. Boonchalermvichian C, Wiwanitkit V. Collection of medical specimen. Chula Med J. 2001; 45: 1079-1089.

7. Wiwanitkit V. Ethics of clinical pathologist. J Med Assoc Thai. 2006;89:2161-2.

8. Wiwanitkit V. Quality control in blood gas analysis. Yasothon Med J 2000; 3: 160-166

9. Ehrmeyer SS, Laessig RH. Point-of-care testing, medical error, and patient safety: a 2007 assessment. Clin Chem Lab Med. 2007;45:766-73.

10. Nichols JH. Quality in point-of-care testing. Expert Rev Mol Diagn. 2003;3:563-72.

11. Carlson DA. Point of care testing: regulation and accreditation. Clin Lab Sci. 1996;9:298-302

Analytical phase for point of care testing

Introduction to analytical **phase**[1]

Analytical phase is the second phase within the laboratory cycle. This is another importhat phase since it is the actual step of analysis within laboratory cycle. Since it directly deals with technical analysis hence any error in this phase is usually relating to analytical procedude and can also affect the whole process of laboratory analysis.

The important concerns on the analytical phase of POCT system is the practitioner. The most important group of medical personnel who perform analysis in the POCT system is the non medical personnel (sometimes the patients). This means the analysis is performed by non expertise. For sure, the accuracy and reliability cannot be as good as those tests performed by medical scientists.

Hence, there is a need for setting of the system to control the quality of the laboratory analysis in analytical phase of PCOT system. The error in this phase is very important and can result in unexpected outcome due to poor patient management.

The author hereby will show some interesting cases.

1. The use of glucometer

    If there is an error in technique, the aberrant high or low blood glucose level can be expected and this futher means the possibility of incorrect adjustment of antidiabetic drug dosage for the patients.

2. The use of blood gas analyzer

    If there is an error in technique, the serious outcome can be expected since the blood gas parameters are the critical parameter for critical care management. Death can be expected.

40

Analytical **technique**[2]

As already mentioned, most of the POCTmeters are usually small and pocket size. The technique is usually based on microfluidics technology. The actual reaction is usually the biochemical rection within the PCOTmeter. Those reactions are the same as standard referencing reactions.

For examples, the important principle of analysis or measurement of some important POCTmeters is hereby listed:

1. Glucometer

   Glucometer makes use of enzymatic technique.

2. Lipidmeter

   Lipidmeter makes use of enzymatic technique.

3. Blood gas analysis

   Blood gas analysis makes use of electrode based technique.

All mentioned methods have to be tested, compared and validated with the standard methods. It is usually seen that the result is parallel in the concordant way. However, it should be noted that the results are usually not the same due to the fact that the POCT system usually uses capillary blood sample whereas the standard system usually uses venous blood sample.

It can be said that the analysis or measurement by POCT tool is easy. The general practice is the use of simple pocket size meter. Using button pressing and minstrip insertion is the basic practice. This allows the general population to use the POCT tool as that in the group with CLEAWAVE guarantee.

However, if there analyzer is the bench-top size, it is usually more complicated and has limited used within the hospital.

Qaulity control for analytical phase for POCT **system**[1, 3 - 4]

In general, quality control is the core principle of laboratory medicine. All laboratory investigations have to pass the acceptable quality control process. The quality control is very important and is the general rule in analytical process (as well as other phases within the laboratory cycle). The quality control in analytical phase implies the standardization of the laboratory. If there is no quality control, it can be said that the laboratory investigation is not reliable and the result is not acceptable for interpretation.

Generally, the quality control has to be

- Routinely performed

- Continuously done

- Scientifically based

- Gently performed

- Recheckable

- Under control of expertise

The quality control in the analytical process of the POCT system is also important. This is the similarity to the general laboratory system.

However, it should be noted that the analysis in POCT system is not within the hand of medical scientist in the central medical laboratory in the hospital. Hence, it cannot be expected for the experience and knowledge of the actual practitioner, nurse and physician. Therefore, it is required to have a specific system to quality control of the analytical phase for POCT system.

The specific characteristic of quality control for analytical phase for POCT system include

- The system is usually not existed.

- It can be implemented by using computer laboratory information management system[5-6].

- It can be controlled by the expertise in the medical laboratory using remote QC technique.

- The basic technique in quality control within the medical laboratory can be used. Levy-Jenning or Westgard rule can be applicable. However, the setting of the acceptable range of QC for the POCT system is usually wider than that of the general laboratory (3 SD, especially those tools for screening pupose)

- There are many specific international standards on the quality control for analytical phase of the POCT system. The good example is that of CAP. It is indicated that the accredited laboratory setting or hospital has to have a specific quality control system for POCT tools[4]

Error in analytical phase of **POCT**[7-8]

Error in laboratory process is the common thing in clinical pathology. In analytical phase, error is detectable. This is also the fact for the POCT system. The error can occur in the analytical phase of POCT system and is an important problem to be solved.

Genreally, the nature of the error in analytical phase of POCT system is identical to that of general laboratory system. There are two main groups of errors, the randomized error and systematic erros.

The use of good quality control system is the core important process to control such erros.

Focusing on the cause of errors in analytical phase of POCT system, the examples are

- Lack of good management system
- Lack of POCT computer laboraoty information management system
- Lack of concern
- Lack of expertise in quality control
- Climate effects (change in temperature and humidity)
- Human error (usually randomized error)
- Instrument error (usually systematic error)

References

1. Wiwanitkit V. Quality management in medical laboratory process. Bangkok: Chulalongkorn University, 2005

2. Prince CP. Point of care testing. BMJ. 2001;322:1285-8.

3. Nichols JH. Quality in point-of-care testing. Expert Rev Mol Diagn. 2003;3:563-72.

4. Carlson DA. Point of care testing: regulation and accreditation. Clin Lab Sci. 1996;9:298-302.

5. Toffaletti J. Wireless POCT data transmission. MLO Med Lab Obs. 2000;32:44-8, 50-1.

6. DuBois JA. Getting to the point: integrating critical care tests in the patient care setting. MLO Med Lab Obs. 2000;32:52-6.

7. Ehrmeyer SS, Laessig RH. Point-of-care testing, medical error, and patient safety: a 2007 assessment. Clin Chem Lab Med. 2007;45:766-73.

8. Meier FA, Jones BA. Point-of-care testing error: sources and amplifiers, taxonomy, prevention strategies, and detection monitors. Arch Pathol Lab Med. 2005;129:1262-7.

Postanalytical phase for point of care testing

Introduction to postanalytical **phase**[1]

Postanalytical phase is the last phase within the laboratory cycle. This is another phase that error can occur. Since it is the final step of laboratory analysis, the error in this step means destruction of the whole process.

Generally, the postanalytical phase covers the validation of the result, result reporting and interpretation of the laboratory results. In general laboratory, this phase requires the communication between the laboratory and the actual user of laboratory result, physician. However, the POCT system reduces the step. The physician who performs the POCT test via POCT tool can get the result and use it at the site of patient treatment (Indeed, this is the aim of developing of the POCT concept).

The characteristics of postanalytical phase for POCT system include:

- Usually lack for laboratory validation

- The result is usually the data shown on the screen of the POCTmeter. Only some POCT meter can print out the result data.

- Backing up of the result is hard if there is no implementation of the computer information management system

- The user, physician incharge, can directly and absuptly use and interpret the investigation result for adjusting the treatment of the patients.

Report of laboratory **result**[1]

Report of the laboratory result is usually the step that can cause the error or delay in general laboratory system. The use of POCT system can help solve the problem. Since the POCT system is designed as a one step service[2] hence it is a good solution of the problem.

There is no need to use the communication technique, media or worker to transport the result from the laboratory to the physician.

For sure, the advantage of this practice is

- Very fast
- Reduce the cause of laboratory result transportation
- Reduce the workload of the laboratory

However, there are many possible problems due to this practice

- Lack for validation of the results
- No rechecking system (since it is a one-stop service with one practitioner)
- There is no format, no specific form of laboratory result report

---

Interpretation of laboratory **result**[1]

In general, the physician incharge is the medical personnel who take the main role in interpretation of laboratory result. The non physician has no role for interpretation of laboratory result. The interpretation of laboratory result means

- the judgement of result that it is normal or not
- the use of result of laboratory analysis for further care of the patient
- answer the hypothesis of illness in the patients

It should be noted that the interpretation result in the POCT system is mainly by the physician who takes the role in POCT analysis hence there are some considerations.

1. The result from the POCT tool will be unreliable if there is no good quality management system, especially for no quality control

2. The result from the POCT tool is not the result from the central medical laboratory. Focusing on the principle of the tool in the POCT system and routine classical laboratory system, there are significant differences. The differences include a) the tool, b) the concept, c) the specimen and etc. It should be noted that the normal value and reference range of the POCT system is not the same as the classical laboratory system. It is not correct to implement the references from classical laboratory to use for the POCT system without setting of new ones.

3. Decision making on the laboratory results should be based on the mentioned normal value and reference range that is specific for POCT system.

4. The record of the laboratory result and interpretation of that result has to clearly indicate the technique of analysis. It has to be clearly demonstrated on the method if the result if from POCT system.

47

Qaulity control for postanalytical phase for POCT **system**[3-4]

The quality control for postanalytical phase for POCT system is also needed. However, the postanalytical phase for POCT system is very short and there is no transportation of laboratory result hence the error rate is very low.

Quality control for postanalytical phase for POCT system has to focus on the randomized error that is cause by human factor. The human error might be due to the reading of the result from the POCTmeter. The reading of the result should be a) single reading, b) recording of the result is needed and c) the POCT computer information management system should be used for further supplementation of the process. This process also results in the transparency in the control of financial system of the laboratory[5].

Waste **management**

Waste management is the necessary process for any laboratory analysis. However, the laboratory analysis according to POCT system required fewer amount of sample comparing to required amount of sample in the case of classical laboratory. Hence, there is not much waste. Generally, there is only the left waste as the strip coded with blood after POCTmeter. The discarding of this waste can follow the general principle for waste management of laboratory wastes and septic materials.

Error in postanalytical phase of **POCT** [6-7]

Error in laboratory process is the common in laboratory analysis and can be seen in any phases of laboratory cycle. In postanalytical phase, error is also detectable. The error can occur in the postanalytical phase of POCT system however it is not as common as that of other phases. The common cause of errors can be

- Incorrect reading of results from the screen of POCTmeter

- Incorrect recording of results from that is displayed within the screen of POCTmeter.

These errors are the randomized errors and results from human errors.

References

1. Wiwanitkit V. Quality management in medical laboratory process. Bangkok: Chulalongkorn University, 2005

2. Prince CP. Point of care testing. BMJ. 2001;322:1285-8.

3. Nichols JH. Quality in point-of-care testing. Expert Rev Mol Diagn. 2003;3:563-72.

4. Carlson DA. Point of care testing: regulation and accreditation. Clin Lab Sci. 1996;9:298-302.

5. Peasrson J. Point-of-care-testing and Clinical Governance. Clin Chem Lab Med. 2006;44:765-7.

6. Ehrmeyer SS, Laessig RH. Point-of-care testing, medical error, and patient safety: a 2007 assessment. Clin Chem Lab Med. 2007;45:766-73.

7. Meier FA, Jones BA. Point-of-care testing error: sources and amplifiers, taxonomy, prevention strategies, and detection monitors. Arch Pathol Lab Med. 2005;129:1262-7.

Point of care testing for blood glucose study

Blood **glucose**[1]

Glucose is the name of a monosaccharide. Glucose is required for living cells of every living things. Glucose is the source of energy and it is an important metabolic intermediate. Glucose is also the energy source of cellular respiration.

The main source of glucose in human beings is the food. There are many foods that pose glucose. When we ingest the food, especially those in the forms of starch and other carbohydrate, the food will be further digested. The digestion will change the carbohydrate into the glucose. The specific enzyme is the amylase. The digestion occurs in two sites, mouth and small intestine. In the mouth, starch will be digested by oral amylase into maltose. In the small intestine, the maltose will be further digested into glucose.

After digestion, the blood glucose will be further absorped for using in the respiratory Krebb's cycle. Generally, the blood glucose level is about 70 - 110 mg%.

The blood glucose within the blood stream is of concern in general medical practice. There are many problems of blood glucsose and the most important one is called diabetes mellitus[2-3]. The important characteristics of diabete mellitus include

- Polyurea

- Polyphagia

- Polydipsia

There are many symptoms and presentations of diabetes mellitus. The common ones include

- No symptom, finding by chance by routine screening

- Has the complete three P's characteristics of diabetes mellitus as already mentioned

- Unexplained weight loss

- Ketoacidosis

- Coma

For the definition, the diabetes mellitus is an endocrine disorder with abnormality of pancrease. The diagnosis is based on the fasting plasma glucose level. The present cut-off value is more than ≥ 126 mg/dl. An alternative diangnosis by hemoglobin A1C more than 7 % is also used in some settings. The diabetes mellitus is the most common endocrine disorder that can be seen in any age and sex.

As described, the best method for diagnosis of diabetes mellitus is the blood test. In general the blood testing for glucose study has to have a specific patient preparation. This process is described as

- Fasting for at least 8 - 14 hours

- Routine eating behavior

- Stop intravenous dextrose administration

- Stop insulin treatment

For the sample collection, these concerns are necessary

- Sodium fluoride tube is requied. This is necessary for prevention of glycolysis.

- In case of emergeny, the clotted blood can be used.

In conclusion, the criteria for diagnosis of diabetes mellitus include

- Fasting blood glucose ≥ 126 mg/dL

- random plama glucose or casual plasma glucose ≥ 200 mg/dL

- hemoglobin A1C ≥ 7 %

- urine glucose (in pregnant subjects at antenatal clinic)

Point of care testing for blood glucose **study**

Generally, the blood glucose study uses the venous blood collection. The blood sample is collected in sodium fluoride tube[4]. It is also recommended for fasting. The routine method for analysis of blood glucose is glucose oxidase method[5]. The routine method for analysis of blood triglyceride is GPO-PAP method. The routine method for analysis of blood LDL cholesterol is PEG-modified enzyme.

Figure 1. Glucose oxidase reaction

glucose + Oxygen in room air --------------------------> Gluconic acid + Hydrogen peroxide

Hydrogen peroxide + Chromogen ----------------------> Oxidized chromogen (blue) + H2O

This is a two-stepped rection. The first step is rather specific however the second reaction is an oxidation reaction with usage of chromogen for formation of color. Hence, it can be easily disturbed by reducing agent such as ascorbic acid or vitamin C. This is the result for possible false positive in measurement.

Focusing on the POCT for blood glucose study, it is not a new approach. Since the POCT for blood glucose study is the first kind of POCT in medicine[6]. The history of glucometer is from its first origin in 1962. It is very useful because of

- the diabetes mellitus is very common hence the use of POCT seems to have high cost utility

- help screening in rural and remote setting

- can be applied for intensive diabetic care

- can be the tools for self adjustment of daily life of diabetic patiens[7-8]

At present, this kind of POCTmeter can be used as tool for self-monitoring[9]. The principle of diabetic self-monitoring is

- based on POCT glucometer that is a CLEAWAVE

- performed at home

- performed by the patient

- recorded of the result by the patient

- data or information on diabetic control will be considerd by physician incharge at each visit

- new remote monitoring system is also available at present

Focusing on the usage procedure of glucometer, it is very simple. The glucometer is usuallt a small pocket size POCTmeter. It can be applied at anty sites. The use of capillary puncture help the general people and layperson perform self punctute to get the blood sample. The recent advent is the use of the new capillary puncture pen. This is very useful and helps decrease the pain sensation of the diabetic patients. The new pen can be adjusted for the depth of puncture. The needle is specifically designed with silicone coat for decreasing pain. The general turnaround time is only 1 minute[7-8].

There are many concerns on the data from the POCT system tool and standard tool for measurement of blood glucose. Mainly, the concern should be one the correlation between the results from the two systems. Wiwanitkit studied the correlation between blood glucose determination by biosensor method and glucose oxidase method and found that the results are comparable[10-11]

However, there are also some important concerns. First, despite the good correlation, the values of the resuls from the two systems are not identical. It should be noted that the result from the capillary sample is usually lower than that of venous sample. This can result in incorrect decision in adjustment of diabetic plan for the diabetic patient. To use the result in following up, it is needed to use the result from the same system for comparison. As already noted, recording of the blood glusoe results has to clearly indicate the analytical technique. The result is due to the principle of testing, oxygen-sensitive glucose oxidase. The result from analysis can be misleaded to the interpretation of hypoglycemia due to the low oxygen in hypotension state. However, at present, there are new developments to find new technique for measurement of blood glucose. This new tool makes use of electrochemical biosensor which is O2-insensitivity that is based on glucose dehydrogenase enzyme[10-11]

Finally, if we focus on medical economics aspect, it is proved that the POCT system is cost effective in actual clinical practice. The good report is that of Wiwanitkit which confirm the cost effective of glucometer comparing to standard method[12]

Other point of care testings for diabetic care[1-2]

In addition to POCT for blood glucose study, there are also other POCTs for diabetic care. Those important tools include

- POCT Microalbumin measurement tool

- POCT Hemoglobin A1C measurement tool

These tools are important for following up and monitoring of diabetic complication. It is recommended that

- Microalbumin testing should be performed annually

- Hemoglobin A1C should be performed every 6 months

There are many available tools for measurement of microalbumin and hemoglobin A1C at present. However, the problem in using of those tools is usually due to the limitation of resource.

References

1. Wiwanitkit V. Laboratory investigation relating to diabetes mellitus. Buddhachinaraj Med J. 2001; 18 (2): 99-103

2. Wiwanitkit V. Laboratory diagnosis for diabetes mellitus. In: Sutheesophon K, Wiwanitkit V, Siritantikorn A. Clinical Pathology. Bangkok: Chulalongkorn University, 2006

3. Diabetes mellitus. Available online at http://hp.anamai.moph.go.th/soongwai/statics/deseas/phyprob/topic004.php

4. Boonchalermvichian C, Wiwanitkit V. Collection of medical specimen. Chula Med J. 2001; 45: 1079-1089.

5. Cooper GR. Methods for determining the amount of glucose in blood. CRC Crit Rev Clin Lab Sci. 1973;4:101-45.

6. Biosensor. Available online at www.gpo.or.th/rdi/html/biosensor.html

7. Glucometer. Available online at www.thailabonline.com/glucomet.htm

8. Glucometer. Available online at www.geocities.com/cddiag/glucomet.htm

9. Prince CP. Point-of-care testing in diabetes mellitus. Clin Chem Lab Med. 2003;41:1213-9.

10. Wiwanitkit V. A comparative study between blood glucose determination by biosensor method and glucose oxidase method. Srinakarind Med J. 2001; 16 : 95-97

11. Wiwanitkit V. Comparative study between glucose determination between capillary biosensor glucose method and standard glucose oxidase method (24th annual scientific meeting on Mahidol's day 22 September 2000). Chiang Mai Med Bull. 2001; 3Suppl : 55.

12. Wiwanitkit V. Cost comparison for glucose testing by point-of-care glucose meter compared with a standard laboratory clinical chemistry analyzer: a patient's perspective from the country of Thailand. POCT. 2007; 6: 118-119.

Point of care testing for lipid study

Blood **lipid**[1 - 2]

Lipid is an important biochemical substance that everyone requires. Fat or lipid is the important food composition. Everyday, we eat lipid food about 60-150 gram. About 90 % of lipid food is in the form of triglyceride. The other parts are the other kinds of lipid such as cholesterol, cholesterol ester, phophoslipid and free fatty acid.

Generally, we ingest lipid food everyday. This is the normal practice of general human beings. After ingestion, the food will be digested and absorped. Focusing on digestion, within mouth and stomach, specific enzyme lipase, linqual lipase and gastric lipase, is avalible. The lipase is the specific enzyme that active in acidic form.

In smalle intestine, the digestion of lipid will be completed with help of emulsifier, the bile acid and bile salt, from biliary canal. After that the absorption of the digested lipid molecule will occur.

The blood lipid within the blood stream is of concern in general medical practice. There are many problems of blood lipid and we called dyslipidemia. The important conditions include

- Hypercholesterolemia

  Hypercholesterolemia is the condition with high level of cholesterol in blood.

- Hypertriglyceridemia

  Hypertriglyceridemia is the condition with high level of cholesterol in blood.

- The importance of hyperlipidemia is because this condition can result in the cardiovascular disease in the future.

  In general, the blood testing for lipid study means the study of 4 components of lipids in blood including[3 - 4]

- Total cholesterol

  It is the general or total form of cholesterol. It contains both high density cholesterol (HDL cholesterol) and low densitiry cholesterol (LDL cholesteroal).

- HDL cholesterol

  This is a good lipid component and can result in the cardiovascular disease. The condition of acute myocardial infarction usually relates with this condition.

- LDL cholesterol

  This is a bad lipid component and can result in the cardiovascular disease. The condition of acute myocardial infarction usually relates with this condition.

- Triglyceride

  This is another bad lipid and can result in the cardiovascular disease. The condition of acute myocardial infarction usually relates with this condition.

In general the blood testing for lipid study has to have a specific patient preparation. This process is described as

- Fasting for at least 8 - 14 hours

- Routine eating behavior

- No other concomitant illness within 3 months

- The blood collection must be in the sitting position (laying position will give lower laboratory results)

Generally, it is recommended for routine screening for blood lipid disorder. Blood lipid study is recommended in

- Any person aged more than 35 years old (screening for total cholesterol)

- Any persone aged more than 35 years old with blood total cholesteroal level more than 240 mg% (screening for total cholesterol, triglyceride and LDL cholesterol)

- Any male aged more than 45 years old and any female aged more than 55 years old (screening for total cholesterol, triglyceride, LDL cholesteroal and HDL cholesterol) [2]

Finally, it should be noted that the level of blood lipid in plasma is lower than in serum. A 4 % differene can be observed.

Point of care testing for lipid **study**

Generally, the lipid study uses the venous blood collection. The blood sample is collected in plain tube. It is also recommended for fasting. The routine method for analysis of blood cholesterol is CHOD-PAP method. The routine method for analysis of blood triglyceride is GPO-PAP method. The routine method for analysis of blood LDL cholesterol is PEG-modified enzyme.

Focusing on the POCT for lipid study, it is a new approach. This is based on the new lipidmeter for POCT system. The lipidmeter uses the capillary blood sample. It is possible to measure total cholesterol and triglyceride. Also, some new POCT meter can measure blood glucsose as well as uric acid at the same single labotatory run. This kind of POCT-meter can be used as tool for self-monitoring similar to glucometer[6].

Focusing on the correlation between blood lipid between classical method and capillary method, Wiwanitkit compared the blood total cholesterol result between those from new biosensor and standard CHOD-PAP method and found a good correlation[7]. Moses et al. also performed a similar study comparing the blood total riglyceride result between those from new biosensor and standard GPO-PAP method method and found the similar concordant result[8]. However, Pimainog et al. noted that the blood total cholesterol and triglyceride levels from capillary blood is significantly higher than those of venous blood. Hence, the cross comparison of lipid profile results between POCT and standard systems has to be careful.

References

1. Digestion and absorption of lipid food. Available online at www.med.cmu.ac.th/dept/biochem/webdept

2. Wiwanitkit V. Screening tests in laboratory medicine : interesting tests and rational use. Chula Med J 2001; 45: 1031-1038.

3. Hyperlipidemia. Available online at http://www.paolosiam.com/b3.html

4. Kovindha S. Hyperlipidemiam and pathology of cardiac vessel. Bull Dept MEd. 2535 ; 17(8) : 580-584.

5. GERTEX - GCT. Available online at www.gertexhealthshop.com/p_GCT.htm

6. Iovine C, Gentile A, Hattemer A, Pacioni D, Riccardi G, Rivellese AA. Self-monitoring of plasma triglyceride levels to evaluate postprandial response to different nutrients. Metabolism. 2004 May;53(5):620-3.

7. Wiwanitkit V. Comparative study between blood cholesterol determination between cholesterol biosensor and standard CHOD-PAP method. Srinagarind Med J. 2001; 16(3): 165-167.

8. Moses RG, Calvert D, Storlien LH. Evaluation of the Accutrend GCT with respect to triglyceride monitoring. Diabetes Care. 1996 Nov;19(11):1305-6.

9. Pimainog Y, Chaiyasut Y, Un-anunt K, Pongsangson P. Evaluation of blood lipids determination by self-monitoring blood lipids mete (Accutrend R GCT). J Med Technol Phys Ther. 2002 ; 14(3): 191-205.

Point of care testing for coagulation study

Blood coagulation **system**

Blood coagulation system is the natural physiological process that corresponds to bleeding. It is considered as a natural defense mechanis. The result is the clot or coagulated blood at the wound site.

The clot is the results from many particles

- Platelet

- Fragmented cells

The mechanism is occurred as the results from thromboplastin from the damaged cells. The thromboplastin will activate a protein in blood stream namely prothrombin to change into enzyme called thrombin. Thrombin will further activet another blood protein namely fibrinoly to change into fibrin which is the weaving network of biosubstances[1]. The final step will result in the blood clot.

Hence, this is the answer to the query why there is no coagulation within blood stream during normal condition without trauma. This is because of there is no thromboplastin hence there will be no thromboplastin, no thrombin and no fibrin at last.

Generally, the coagulation system will have two important kinds of reaction. The two kinds are called intrinsic pathway and extrinsic pathway[2]. These two pathways simulataneously occur in natural condition. When one examines the problem in coagulation system, the concern on both intrinsic and extrinsic pathways is needed.

Problem on blood **coagulation**

There are two main important problems of blood coagulation.

1. Increased bleeding tendency [3-4]

   Increased bleeding tendency is an important disorder that might be the result of the abnormality in blood coagulation system. This can be either vascular, platelet or coagulation factors.

   - Vascular cause
     - Dengue hemorrhagic fever
     - Fragile blood vessel
   - Platelet cause
     - Dengue hemorrhagic fever
     - Aplastic anemia
     - Leukemia
     - SLE
     - ITP
   - Coagulation factors cause
     - Hemophilia
     - Cirrhosis
     - Renal failure
     - Venomous snake bite

2. Hypercoagulable state [5]

   Hypercoagulable state directly relates to thrombosis. The thrombosis is the result from the clotted particle called thrombus. Within the thrombus, there are many compositions including to platelet, white blood cell, red blood cell, fibrin and etc.

   Thrombus can be seen at many sites in vivo such as venous blood vessel, arterial blood vessel as well as heart.

   The effect of thrombus can be in many form such as rupture, infarction and etc.

POCT for coagulation **study**

Generally, the coagulation study in laboratory medicine is a group of widelty used hematology test in medical practice. It is useful for the management of the patient with coagulation problem.

In general, the two most common tests in general practice are PT and PTT. The two main aims of testings are a) diagnosis of abnormality of blood coagulation and b) following up of the drug treatment that has effect of blood coagulation. The quality control of these tests is very important[6]. The study by Wiwanitkit noted that there are a considerable number of errors in coagulation testing[7].

The use of POCT for coagulation study in the present day is usually for the second aim, therapeutic drug monitoring for anticoagulation therapy. In general, anticoagulant therapy, there are two main kinds of anticoagulant drugs[8]

1. heparin [8-9]

   Heparin is a non oral form of anticoagulant drug. The monitoring is generally by PTT

2. coumarin[10]

   Coumarin is an oral form of anticoagulant drug. It is widely used at present. The monitoring is usuauly via PT. However, since there are variation of PT value due to the reagent in the reaction[11], the new standardized parameter namely International Normalized Ratio (INR) must be used. Generall, INR can be derived by this formula

$$INR = (patient\ PT/mean\ normal\ PT)^{ISI}$$

   The normal value of INR is about 0.9 □□□ 1.1.

Table 1. The target INR value for coumarin therapy12.

Aim	Target INR value
General prevention	2.0-3.0
General treatment	2.0-3.0
Case with recurrent systemic embolism	2.0-3.5
Case on mechanical prosthetic valves	2.0-3.5

The investigation on coagulation system via the POCT system can be done at present using the POCTmeter. The small POCTmeters are available and very useful in clinical practice. There are many reports confirming that the PT and INR results from POCT system are comparable to those results from classical reference methods.

References

1. Hemker HC, Al Dieri R, De Smedt E, Beguin S. Thrombin generation, a function test of the haemostatic-thrombotic system. Thromb Haemost. 2006 Nov;96(5):553-61.

2. Chuansumrit A. Coagulation process. Available online at □□□ http://www.ramacme.org/articles/3-16-207-2108-0411-01/3-16-207-2108-0411-01-003.asp

3. Carnelli V, Dozzi M, Gibelli M, Giovanniello A, Riva F, Seidita C, Stucchi C. Children with hemorrhagic diathesis: correct diagnostic and therapeutic approach. Pediatr Med Chir. 1990;12:1-13.

4. Lillicrap D, Nair SC, Srivastava A, Rodeghiero F, Pabinger I, Federici AB. Laboratory issues in bleeding disorders. Haemophilia. 2006 Jul;12 Suppl 3:68-75.

5. Circulatory Disturbances. Available online at http://202.28.92.162/mediacenter/mediacenter-uploads/libs/html/1186/gp4.htm

6. Wiwanitkit V. ISO 15189, some comments on its application in the coagulation laboratory. Blood Coagul Fibrinolysis. 2004;15:613-7.

7. Rejection of specimens for prothrombin time and relating pre-analytical factors in blood collection. Blood Coagul Fibrinolysis. 2002;13:371-2.

8. Tositarattana T. Thromobis and antithrombosis. Available online at http://www.ams.cmu.ac.th/depts/clinmcrs/b16.doc

9. Wiwanitkit V. Using heparin tube for clinical chemistry. Songkhanagarind Med J. 2003; 21: 217-222

10. Deckert FW. Coumarin anticoagulants: a review of some current research areas. South Med J. 1974;67:1191-202.

11. Wiwanitkit V. Comparison of prothrombin time determination from different reagents by automated and semi-automated methods. Songkhanagarind Med J. 2001; 19: 13-16.

12. WAFARIN... How to use? Available online at www.vajira.ac.th/pharmacy/Data/newsdrug/newsdrug.doc

Blood gas analysis and oint of care testing

Introduction to blood gas **analysis**

Blood gas analysis is an important laboratory analysis.[1][2] This laboratory test is classified as the critical parameter. Arterial blood gas analysis is widely used. This specific test is important for treatment and diagnosis of the critical illed patients.

The general usage of blood gas analysis is for

- Assessment of oxygenation in blood
- Assessment of ventilation
- Assessment of acid base and pH within blood

The general usage of blood gas analysis is for critical care. The examples of usage are

- Patients in intensive care unit
- Patients on oxygen therapy
- Patient on anesthesia procedure
- Patient with respiratory failure
- Patient with disturbance on acid base status
  - Severe diarrhea
  - Renal failure
  - Intoxication

The arterial blood analysis is an actual testing for critical care testing. It is used in many branches of medicine including

- Chest medicine
- Neurosurgery
- Neonatology
- Anesthesiology

Interpretation of blood gas analysis is necessary in laboratotry medicine. If it is not possible to interprete, it will be useless.

In the blood gas analysis report, there will be these important informations[2-3]

1. pO2

   The normal value is 80 -100 mmHg. This parameter is for assessment of oxygenation.The low value is called hypoxemia. This value is directly measured by the blood gas analyzer.

2. pCO2

   The normal value is 35 - 45 mmHg. This parameter is for assessment of ventilation. The low value is called hyperventilation and the high value is called hypoventilation. This value is directly measured by the blood gas analyzer.

3. pH

   The normal value is 7.35 - 7.45. The low value is called acidemia and the high value is called alkalemia. This value is directly measured by the blood gas analyzer.

In interpretation of blood gas analysis, the physician inchage needs to interpret the parameters in the report form as well as the medical history, physical examination and other laboratory parameters.

Table 1. Interpretation of arterial blood gas.

Condition	pH	pCO2	HCO3
Normal	73.5-7.45	35-45	22-26
Respiratory acidodis	Decrease	Increase	Normal
Respiratory alkalosis	Decrease	Decrease	Normal
Metabolic acidosis	Decrease	Normal	Decrease
Metabolic alkalosis	Increase	Normal	Increase

POCT for arterial blood gas **analysis**

Arterial blood ga analysis is the measurement of gas within arterial blood. It can relate to respiratory and metabolic disorders. It helps assess the pH within blood referring to acid and based status. Also, it helps tell the ventilation and oxygenation status.

This test is an emergency test hence the rapid turnaround time is very important. Hence, the concept of POCT can be implemented for the blood gas analysis. The reasons are

- arterial blood gas is the test that required short turnaround time

- it should give the result at the patient care site

- it should help reduce the transportation of specimen to reduce error

For the analysis, the specific blood gas analyzer can be used. This is the tool that can be applied as POCTmeter.

The samples for the blood gas analyzer can be

1. arterial blood sample

   This sample should be gently collected as previously described in the previous chapter. This is the standard sample type for arterial blood gas analysis in general practice. The most common site for sample collection is radial artery. If there is no palpating pulse, the puncture is contraindicated. Also, it is needed to apply the pressure at the puncture site after arterial blood collection. Observation of the complications especially for hematoma formation after arterial puncture is required[2-3].

2. capillary blood sample

   This sample is used in some cases. The incidation is for the pediatric population that arterial blood collection is considerd too harmful to do. The special preparation as warming the collection size to get the finalized arterialized capillary blood.

Focusing on the technique of analysis, the analyzer uses only a few samples, less than 90 microliters.

- pH , PCO_2 and PO_2 in blood is directly measured via electrode

- Baromatic Pressure is directly measured via electrode

- Total CO_2 , Bicarbonate , Base Excess , Oxygen Content , Oxygen , Saturation and PO_2 (A/a) is calculated from the automatic microprocessor function within the arterial blood gas analyzer.

The results are generally displayed on the screen which is vacuum fluorescent size and can be printed out in paper form. In addition, the arterial blood gas analyzer has automatic washing system for cleasing. The electrode is usually a ready maintenance electrode[4].

Due to the advent in technology, there are many new arterial blood gas analyzers at present. Some new analyzers are very small and can be useful for actual usage. However, these analyzers usually have higher cost comparing to the standard classical analyzer[5].

In addition, the new generation of arterial blood gas analyzer usually has the ability to analyzer additional laboratory parameters especially for blood electrolyte. Since the basic principle for analysis of blood electrolyte is the electrode technique hence it is usually included in the new generation of arterial blood gas analyzers.

The important electrolytes to be measure include

- Sodium

- Potassium

- Chloride

References

1. Vichitvejpaisarn P. Blood gas analysis. 2^{nd}ed. Bangkok: TA living, 1997: 121 – 65.

2. Wiwanitkit V. Blood gas analysis. Available at http://cai.md.chula.ac.th/lesson/lesson4409/

3. Wiwanitkit V. Quality control in blood gas analysis. Yasothorn Med J. 2000; 2: 160-166.

4. Larppongtorn V, Apakupakul N. Accuracy of i-STAT compared to ABL-3 in estimating pH, pCO2 and pO2 of blood gas. Songkla Med J 2001; 19: 25-30

5. Boemke W, Krebs MO, Rossaint R. Blood gas analysis. Anaesthesist. 2004;53:471-92

Point of care testing for thyroid disease

Introduction to thyroid
disease

Thyroid is an important endocrine of human beings. It locates at the anterior neck. This is a small glad but it is very important. The main functions of thyroid gland include:

- Control of energetic metabolism within human body

- Control of calcium metabolism

  The thyroid gland is a good example of endocrine gland. It secrets two main kinds of hormone

- Thyroid hormone

  Thyroid hormone is the main hormone from thyroid cell. It takes main role in control of energetic metabolism within human body

- Calcitonin

  This hormone is secreted from C cell in thyroid gland. Calcitonin plays important role in calcium metabolism regulation. Its function is reduction of blood calcium.

Interestingly, the control of thyroid activity is by the feedback loop from anterior pituitary. The control is via the thyroid stimulating hormone (TSH). The excessive or too high level of thyroid hormone will decrease the level of TSH. The too low level of thyroid hormone will induce increased secretion of TSH vise versa.

There are many abnormalities of thyroid. The common diseases include

1. Hyper and hypothyroidism

2. Tumor of thyroid

3. Thyroiditis

Of several diseases, the important one is the hyper and hypothyroidism. These conditions are more common than others. Hyper and hypothyroidism are the actual condition in general practice.

Why the POCT is useful for management of thyroid **disease**?

Since the hyper and hypothyroidism are common in general practice, it is no doubt that there are many laboratory investigations for these two disorders. The common laboratory investigations is called thyroid function test.

The thyroid function test includes

- T3:

  T 3 is the total hormone in triiodo-form secreted from thyroid gland.

- Free T3

  Free T3 is the active form of T3.

- T4:

  T 4 is the total hormone with four iodine molecules secreted from thyroid gland.

- Free T4:

  Free T4 is the active form of T4.

- TSH:

  As already noted, TSH is the regulatory hormone from anterior pituitary gland.

Of all five tests, the three common tests at present are TSH, free T3 and free T4.

Generally, the laboratory tests for these parameters need blood collection and the analysis by autormated clinical chemistry analyzer. This means it has to take a considerable amount of time. In general, the patient has to have a previous blood collection and wait for result.

However, the problem of waiting can be expected in some cases. These are the good examples:

- In screening for congenital hypothyrodism

  The congenital hypothyroidism is the condition with the lack of thyroid hormone in the neonate. This condition is problematic. Since the thyroid hormone is necessary for neurological development of the infant and lack of thyroid hormone means permanent brain dysfunction, it is needed to screen and early detect of the disorder. The key point is the fact that there is an effective drug, thyroid hormone extract that can effectively prevent the sequele from congenital deficit of thyroid hormone.

- In case of thyroid storm

  The thyroid storm is an actual emergency in medicine. This means the severity and life threatening condition. The diagnosis of this condition has to be fast. The rapid test is needed. Since the treatment is usually effective, the core concept for management is early diagnosis.

The solution from those mentioned problems can be derived from the use of POCT tool.

POCT tools for thyroid **diseases**

There are many kinds of POCT at present. However, there are not many specific tools for thyroid disease. An important tool is the TSHmeter. This kind of POCT tool can be applicable for usage in detection of hypothyroidism in both infant and adult population.

The use of TSHmeter helps fasten the process of screening for hypothyroidism in both infant and adult groups[1]. The problem of the present system that uses venous or capillary blood can be solved. At first, the system requires very few amount of blood sample and can give the result within few minutes. Second, the problem of specimen collection on filter paper and transportation of sample to reference laboratory in general practice for routine screening for neonatal hypothyroidism can be effectively solved.

The principle of TSHmeter is usually based on the immunological method and the reading of the result is based on the general POCTmeter concept. The result can be read either in qualitative or quantitative fashions. In real clinical practice, the use of TSHmeter is confirmed for its utility in screening program for finding congenital hypothyroidism. In a recent report in Uganda, Ehrenkranz et al. concluded that "Assessing neonatal TSH levels in developing countries with a TSH assay method suitable for field use can be successfully used to screen for congenital hypothyroidism and to indirectly assess a population's iodine status[2]."

However, at present, the TSHmeter is not routinely used due to many facts. First, the cost of the TSHmeter is expensive and this might not be affordable for many poor setting in the developing countries. Second, the TSHmeter can only provide the result for TSH. It cannot provide the data of free T3 and free T4 that is generally used for following up process of hyper and hypothyroidism cases.

Another kind of analyzer is the dry chemistry form analyzer. This kind of analyzer can analyze for many clinical chemistry parameters including TSH and T3, T4. This might be helpful for using as tool for following up of hypo and hyperthyroidism cases. Also, this kind of POCT analyzer can be used for other disorders. However, an important concern is its nature of dry chemistry analyzer. Some setting might not use it as a POCTmeter but as a dry chemistry analyzer in central laboratory. This means reduction of usefulness in reduction of turnaround time. In the study of Grodzinsky et al., up to 2 days of turnaround time can be observed[3]. How to encourage the correct usage of POCT tool is the thing to be discussed.

Finally, it should be noted that there is also the specific POCT assay for autoantibody detection which is useful for management of autoimmune thyroid diseases such as Graves disease. At present, POCT assays for autoantibodies to thyroid peroxidase and to thyroglobulin are available. Burne et al. noted that this kind of POCT meter was useful for prediction of postpartum thyroiditis and the development of interferon-alpha-related thyroid disease[4].

As a conclusion, POCT tool for thyroid disease is an actual advent in the development of endocrinology laboratory at present[5].

References

1. Duntas LH, Koutras DA. Application of ThyroChek in the assessment of the various degrees of hypothyroidism. Thyroid. 1999;9:847-8.

2. Ehrenkranz J, Fualal J, Ndizihiwe A, Clarke I, Alder S. Neonatal age and point of car-eTSH testing in the monitoring of iodine deficiency disorders: findings from western Uganda. Thyroid. 2011;21:183-8.

3. Grodzinsky E, Wirehn AB, Fremner E, Haglund S, Larsson L, Persson LG, Borgquist L. Point-of-care testing has a limited effect on time to clinical decision in primary health care. Scand J Clin Lab Invest. 2004;64:547-51.

4. Burne P, Mitchell S, Rees Smith B. Point-of-care assays for autoantibodies to thyroid peroxidase and to thyroglobulin. Thyroid. 2005;15:1005-10.

5. Lepage R, Albert C. Fifty years of development in the endocrinology laboratory. Clin Biochem. 2006;39:542-57.